101 SMOOTHIE RECIPES

Boost Your Immune System | Gain Strength | Accelerate Weight Loss | Detoxify Your Body

Copyright © 2016

By

MFRC Publishing

N.S. NASH

Everyone Love Smoothies and it's so easy to make. Smoothies are heart-healthy drink and help to boost your immune system, gain strength, accelerate weight loss, and it detoxifies your body.

Smoothies are the best way to get instant energy and are the fastest meal to make. Fruits and vegetables are nutritious in any form. They can provide all the nutrients you need just add the fruits and vegetables you want and blend it.

Weight Loss: A banana smoothie makes a perfect fit for your weight loss diet. Bananas are naturally sweet and can help curb your sweet tooth for that afternoon sugar craving. A regular banana has around 90 calories and is rich in a mineral electrolyte called potassium. Bananas have a small amount of vitamin A, adding a banana to your diet also helps keep your eyes healthy.

Detoxification: Eating a diet rich in vegetables and fruits as part of an overall healthy diet may reduce risk for heart disease, including heart attack and stroke. Research shows that they may also protect against certain types of cancers. Fruits and veggies provide fiber to your body that helps fill you up and keeps your digestive system happy. Fiber may reduce the risk of heart disease, obesity, and type-2 diabetes. Eating vegetables and fruits rich in potassium may lower blood pressure, and may also reduce the risk of developing kidney stones and help to decrease bone loss. They are naturally low in calories and may help reduce the risk of many diseases including, heart disease, high blood pressure and some cancers. They are rich in vitamins and minerals that help you feel healthy and energized.

101 SMOOTHIE RECIPES: These are delicious healthy smoothie recipes which will boost your immune system, gain strength, accelerate weight loss, and it detoxifies your body.

It's near impossible to screw up a smoothie. Throw any combination of milk, fruit, nuts, and other goodies into a blender and presto: You've got drinkable meal.

Note: use blender with ice crushing ability.

Caution: avoid any ingredient(s) you are allergic to.

Find out how to accelerate weight loss, gain strength, and boost your immune system with 101 smoothie recipes!

Health Benefits

- *Reduce bad cholesterol*
- *Get a healthier heart*
- *Control your weight*
- *Detoxify your liver*
- *Boost your immune system*
- *Reducing your risk of stroke*
- *Overcome depression*
- *Sustain your blood sugar*
- *Against muscle cramps during workouts and night time leg cramps*
- *Strengthen your blood*
- *Aid digestion*
- *Can maintain the body temperature*
- *Improve immune system*
- *Help you quit smoking*
- *Accelerate weight loss*

Strawberry-Banana-Pineapple Smoothie

Ingredients:

- 1 cup pineapple juice
- 1 cup low-fat vanilla yogurt or 1 cup low-fat vanilla frozen yogurt
- 1 cup frozen strawberries, partially thawed
- 2 ripe medium bananas, peeled

Directions:

Combine ingredients in blender and blend until smooth. Pour smoothie into tall glass and serve.

Winter Greens Smoothie

Ingredients:

- 1/4 cup carrot juice
- 1/2 cup orange juice
- 1 cup spinach
- 1 cup roughly chopped kale, ribs removed
- 4 small broccoli florets, sliced and frozen
- 1 banana, peeled, sliced, and frozen
- 1 apple, cored and roughly chopped

Directions:
Combine ingredients in blender and blend until smooth. Pour smoothie into tall glass and serve.

Tropical Green Smoothie

Ingredients:

- 12 oz water, milk, or yogurt
- 2 scoops vanilla flavored protein powder
- 1/2 banana
- 1 cup of pineapple
- 1 cup of spinach
- 1 tbsp of ground flax
- 2 tbsp of unsweetened coconut flakes
- 1/2 cup plain yogurt or vegan alternative

Directions:

Combine ingredients in blender and blend until smooth. Pour smoothie into tall glass and serve.

Apple-Banana Smoothie

Ingredients:

- 1 apple
- 1/2 frozen banana
- 1/4 cup cashews
- 1 scoop hemp protein
- 2 pitted dates
- 1 cup almond milk
- 1 teaspoon apple pie spice
- 3 ice cubes

Directions:
Combine ingredients in blender and blend until smooth. Pour smoothie into tall glass and serve.

Papaya Smoothie

Ingredients:

- 2 cups chopped peeled seeded papayas
- 1 cup chilled pineapple juice
- ½ cup milk
- ½ cup sliced banana
- 4 ice cubes
- 1 tablespoon honey
- 2 teaspoons fresh lime juice

Directions:
Combine ingredients in blender and blend until smooth. Pour smoothie into tall glass and serve.

Kale, Apple & Lime Smoothie

Ingredients:

- 2 large handfuls of kale
- 2 cups apple juice
- Juice of 1/2 a lime
- 1 banana
- Handful of ice as needed

Directions:
Combine ingredients in blender and blend until smooth. Pour smoothie into tall glass and serve.

Apple Pie Smoothie

- 4 ice cubes
- 1 banana
- 1 cup unsweetened applesauce
- ½ cup no-sugar-added nonfat vanilla yogurt
- ½ cup apple juice
- 1 tablespoon Splenda sugar substitute (or sugar)
- ¼ teaspoon ground nutmeg
- ½ teaspoon ground cinnamon
- ¼ teaspoon ground allspice

Directions:
Combine ingredients in blender and blend until smooth. Pour smoothie into tall glass and serve.

Cantaloupe, Berry & Pineapple Smoothie

Ingredients:

- 1 cup cranberry juice
- 1 cup cantaloupe, diced
- 1 cup blackberry
- 1 cup pineapple, diced

Directions:
Combine ingredients in blender and blend until smooth. Pour smoothie into tall glass and serve.

Green Raspberry Smoothie

Ingredients:

- Handful raspberries
- 1/2 small tart green apple
- Large handful spinach
- 1 tablespoon raw almond butter
- 1/2 cup unsweetened light coconut milk
- 1/2 cup coconut water
- Splash vanilla extract
- Ice cubes (optional)

Directions:
Combine ingredients in blender and blend until smooth. Pour smoothie into tall glass and serve.

Tropical Fruit Smoothie

Ingredients:

- 1/4 cup (60 mL) fresh or canned pineapple chunks
- 1/4 cup (60 mL) fresh mango chunks
- 2 fresh or frozen strawberries, hulled
- 1 cup (250 mL) plain low-fat soy milk
- 1 Tbsp (15 mL) lime juice

Directions:
Combine ingredients in blender and blend until smooth. Pour smoothie into tall glass and serve.

Go Green Smoothie

Ingredients:

- 2 cups Spinach
- 1/2 cucumber
- 1/4 head of celery
- 1/2 bunch parsley
- 1 bunch of mint
- 3 carrots
- 2 apples
- 1/4 orange, 1/4 lime, 1/4 lemon
- 1/4 pineapple

Directions:
Combine ingredients in blender and blend until smooth. Pour smoothie into tall glass and serve.

Apple & Great Grains Smoothie

Ingredients:

- 12 oz water, milk, or yogurt
- 2 scoops vanilla flavored protein
- 1 apple, core removed, and sliced into wedges
- 1 cup of spinach
- 2 tbsp of almonds
- 1/4 cup of uncooked oats
- Ice as needed
- Cinnamon to taste

Directions:
Combine ingredients in blender and blend until smooth. Pour smoothie into tall glass and serve.

Baked Apple Smoothie

Ingredients:

- 12 oz water, milk, or yogurt
- 2 scoops vanilla flavored protein powder
- 1 apple, core removed, and sliced into wedges
- 1 cup of spinach
- 1 tbsp of almonds
- 1 tbsp of ground flax
- 1 tbsp of sesame seeds
- Cinnamon to taste
- Ice as needed

Directions:
Combine ingredients in blender and blend until smooth. Pour smoothie into tall glass and serve.

Hawaiian Smoothie

Ingredients:

- 1 cup chopped fresh pineapple
- 1/2 cup chopped peeled papaya
- 1/4 cup guava nectar (see Tip)
- 1 tablespoon lime juice
- 1 teaspoon grenadine
- 1/2 cup ice

Directions:
Combine ingredients in blender and blend until smooth. Pour smoothie into tall glass and serve.

Apple-Spinach Smoothie

Ingredients:

- 2 cups spinach
- 1 chopped peeled apple
- 1/2 cup silken tofu
- 1/4 cup each soy milk and orange juice
- 1 tablespoon each wheat germ
- Honey and lemon juice
- 1 cup ice

Directions:
Combine ingredients in blender and blend until smooth. Pour smoothie into tall glass and serve.

Creamy Pineapple Smoothie

Ingredients:

- 2 cups chopped pineapple
- 1/2 cup cottage cheese
- 1/4 cup milk
- 2 teaspoons honey
- 1/4 teaspoon vanilla
- a pinch each of nutmeg and salt
- 2 cups ice

Directions:
Combine ingredients in blender and blend until smooth. Pour smoothie into tall glass and serve.

Peanut Butter–Apple Smoothie

Ingredients:

- 1 chopped peeled apple
- 3 tablespoons creamy peanut butter
- 2 tablespoons flaxseeds
- 1 1/2 cups soy milk
- 1 1/2 cups ice
- Honey to taste

Directions:
Combine ingredients in blender and blend until smooth. Pour smoothie into tall glass and serve.

Tofu Tropic Smoothie

Ingredients:

- 2 cups diced frozen mango
- 11/2 cups pineapple juice
- 3/4 cup silken tofu
- 1/4 cup lime juice
- 1 teaspoon freshly grated lime zest

Directions:
Combine ingredients in blender and blend until smooth. Pour smoothie into tall glass and serve.

Pineapple Watermelon Tango Smoothie

Ingredients:

- 1 cup pineapple, diced
- 1 cup watermelon, diced
- ½ cup orange juice
- 100 g frozen yoghurt (optional)
- ½ cup ice cube (optional)

Directions:
Combine ingredients in blender and blend until smooth. Pour smoothie into tall glass and serve.

Pineapple Orange Smoothie

Ingredients:

- 12 ounces orange juice
- ½ cup pineapple chunk, drained
- 1 ¼ cups low-fat vanilla yogurt

Directions:
Combine ingredients in blender and blend until smooth. Pour smoothie into tall glass and serve.

Peachy Pineapple Smoothie

Ingredients:

- 28 ounces of sliced peaches
- ½ cup pineapple juice, chilled
- ¼ cup sugar
- 1 pint vanilla ice cream, softened

Directions:
Combine ingredients in blender and blend until smooth. Pour smoothie into tall glass and serve.

Mojito Smoothie

Ingredients:

- 1 1/2 cups nut milk or coconut water
- 3 tablespoons hemp seeds
- 1/2-1 teaspoon spirulina
- 4 tablespoons lime juice
- 1 avocado
- 1 frozen banana
- 2 pitted dates
- Handful fresh mint leaves (20-25 leaves)

Directions:
Combine ingredients in blender and blend until smooth. Pour smoothie into tall glass and serve.

Chocolate Sunbutter Cup Smoothie

Ingredients:

- 3 tablespoons cacao powder
- 2 tablespoons sunflower seed butter
- 1/2 cup packed spinach
- 3 dates
- 1/4 avocado
- 1 1/2 cups almond or coconut milk (frozen into ice cubes, if desired)
- Maca powder (optional)
- For garnish (optional): Coconut flakes, Cacao nibs, Hemp seeds, Raspberries

Directions:

Combine ingredients in blender and blend until smooth. Pour smoothie into tall glass and serve.

Raspberry-Avocado Smoothie

Ingredients:

- 1 avocado, peeled and pitted
- 3/4 cup orange juice
- 3/4 cup raspberry juice
- 1/2 cup frozen raspberries (not thawed)

Directions:
Combine ingredients in blender and blend until smooth. Pour smoothie into tall glass and serve.

Good Green Tea Smoothie

Ingredients:

- 3 cups frozen white grapes
- 2 packed cups baby spinach
- 11/2 cups strong brewed green tea, cooled
- 1 medium ripe avocado
- 2 teaspoons honey

Directions:
Combine ingredients in blender and blend until smooth. Pour smoothie into tall glass and serve.

Berry Cherry Smoothie

Ingredients:

- 1/2 cup frozen cherries
- 8 oz water
- 1/2 cup chopped raw beets
- 1/2 cup frozen strawberries
- 1/2 cup frozen blueberries
- 1/2 banana
- 1 scoop chocolate whey protein
- 1 tbsp ground flaxseed

Directions:
Combine ingredients in blender and blend until smooth. Pour smoothie into tall glass and serve.

Blueberry Breakfast Smoothie

Ingredients:

- 1 cup blueberries
- 1/2 banana
- 1 1/2 scoops protein powder
- 2 tbsp walnuts
- 2 tbsp oats
- 1 tbsp chia seeds

Directions:

Combine ingredients in blender and blend until smooth. Pour smoothie into tall glass and serve.

Frozen Fruit Smoothie

Ingredients:

- 2 cups of orange juice
- 1 cup of frozen berries
- 1 banana
- 1 tbsp chia seeds
- 3 tbsp rolled oats

Directions:

Combine ingredients in blender and blend until smooth. Pour smoothie into tall glass and serve.

Strawberry Mango Spring Smoothie

Ingredients:

- 1 cup coconut milk
- 1 banana, peeled, sliced, and frozen
- 1 mango, skinned and chunked
- 5 large strawberries, hulled

Directions:
Combine ingredients in blender and blend until smooth. Pour smoothie into tall glass and serve.

Strawberry Banana Kefir Smoothie

Ingredients:

- 1 cup plain low-fat kefir
- 2 tbsp walnuts
- 1 cup chopped strawberries
- 1 banana
- 1 scoop vanilla whey protein
- Water as needed

Directions:
Combine ingredients in blender and blend until smooth. Pour smoothie into tall glass and serve.

Spinach Flax Smoothie

Ingredients:

- 1/2 cup vanilla yogurt
- 1 cup milk
- 1 tablespoon natural peanut butter
- 2 cups spinach
- 1 frozen banana
- 3 strawberries
- 1 teaspoon flaxseed

Directions:
Combine ingredients in blender and blend until smooth. Pour smoothie into tall glass and serve.

Strawberry Banana Smoothie

Ingredients:

- 12 oz water, milk, or yogurt
- 2 scoops vanilla or strawberry flavored protein powder
- 1 banana
- 1 cup of frozen strawberries
- 1 cup of spinach
- 2 tbsp of ground flax

Directions:
Combine ingredients in blender and blend until smooth. Pour smoothie into tall glass and serve.

Strawberry Smoothie

Ingredients:

- 1 cup frozen strawberries
- 1 cup milk
- ¼ cup sugar
- 1 banana
- 8 to 10 ice cubes

Directions:
Combine ingredients in blender and blend until smooth. Pour smoothie into tall glass and serve.

Fruit & Oat Smoothie

Ingredients:

- 1 cup quartered strawberries
- 1 sliced banana
- 1/4 cup raw almonds
- 1/2 cup old-fashioned oats
- 1 cup low-fat vanilla yogurt
- 1 teaspoon maple syrup

Directions:

Combine ingredients in blender and blend until smooth. Pour smoothie into tall glass and serve.

Banana Cranberry & Orange Smoothie

Ingredients:

- ½ cup orange juice
- ½ cup cranberry juice
- 1 banana

Directions:

Combine ingredients in blender and blend until smooth. Pour smoothie into tall glass and serve.

Berry-Flaxseed Smoothie

Ingredients:

- 2 tablespoons whole flaxseeds
- 1/2 cup orange juice
- 1/2 cup nonfat vanilla yogurt
- 1 cup unsweetened frozen mixed berries or blueberries
- 1 small banana, sliced

Directions:
Combine ingredients in blender and blend until smooth. Pour smoothie into tall glass and serve.

Pomegranate Berry Smoothie

Ingredients:

- 2 cups frozen mixed berries
- 1 cup pomegranate juice
- 1 medium banana
- 1/2 cup nonfat cottage cheese
- 1/2 cup water

Directions:
Combine ingredients in blender and blend until smooth. Pour smoothie into tall glass and serve.

Spinach & Strawberry Smoothie

Ingredients:

- 1/2 cup (125 mL) low-fat vanilla yogurt
- 2 cups (500 mL) water
- 1 medium banana
- 1 cup (250 mL) sliced strawberries
- 2 cups (500 mL) chopped fresh spinach, lightly packed
- Honey or maple syrup to taste (optional)

Directions:
Combine ingredients in blender and blend until smooth. Pour smoothie into tall glass and serve.

Banana-Agave Smoothie

Ingredients:

- 1 cup plain fat-free yogurt
- 1/3 cup fresh or frozen blueberries, thawed
- 2 teaspoons light-colored agave nectar
- 1 chilled sliced ripe banana

Directions:
Combine ingredients in blender and blend until smooth. Pour smoothie into tall glass and serve.

Banana Java Smoothie

Ingredients:

- 1 cup coffee
- 1 cup unsweetened almond milk
- 1 scoop vanilla whey protein powder
- 1 banana, 1/4 cup oats
- 1 tablespoon raw cocoa powder
- 1 tablespoon chia seeds
- 1/8 teaspoon ground cardamom

Directions:
Combine ingredients in blender and blend until smooth. Pour smoothie into tall glass and serve.

Peachy Oat Smoothie

Ingredients:

- 1 peach
- 2 cups spinach
- 2 tablespoons chia seeds
- 1/2 frozen banana
- 1/2 orange
- 1/4 cup plain yogurt
- 1 date (optional)

Directions:
Combine ingredients in blender and blend until smooth. Pour smoothie into tall glass and serve.

Chocolate-Banana Smoothie

Ingredients:

- 1 cup frozen sliced banana (about 1 large)
- 2 cups 1% low-fat chocolate milk
- 2/3 cup fat-free,
- No-sugar-added chocolate fudge ice cream
- Chocolate shavings (optional)

Directions:

Combine ingredients in blender and blend until smooth. Pour smoothie into tall glass and serve.

Chocolate Espresso Protein Smoothie

Ingredients:

- 1 banana, chunked and frozen
- 1 scoop chocolate protein powder
- 1 tsp instant coffee grounds {or 1/2 cup brewed coffee, chilled}
- 1 tsp unsweetened cocoa powder
- 1 tsp coconut palm sugar (optional)
- 1 cup coconut milk (or other milk)
- 1/2 cup ice (optional)

Directions:
Combine ingredients in blender and blend until smooth. Pour smoothie into tall glass and serve.

Mocha Breakfast Smoothie

Ingredients:

- 12 oz cold black coffee
- 1 frozen banana
- 2 scoops chocolate whey protein powder
- 1 tbsp unsweetened cocoa
- Handful of walnuts
- 1 cup of ice

Directions:

Combine ingredients in blender and blend until smooth. Pour smoothie into tall glass and serve.

Banana-Cocoa Soy Smoothie

Ingredients:

- 1 banana
- 1/2 cup silken tofu
- 1/2 cup soymilk
- 2 tablespoons unsweetened cocoa powder
- 1 tablespoon honey

Directions:

Combine ingredients in blender and blend until smooth. Pour smoothie into tall glass and serve.

Coconut Lime Smoothie

Ingredients:

- 1/2 sliced banana
- 1/2 diced mango
- 1/3 cup coconut milk
- 1 lime, zested and juiced
- Pinch ground cardamom
- 3 ice cubes

Directions:
Combine ingredients in blender and blend until smooth. Pour smoothie into tall glass and serve.

Pumpkin Smoothie

Ingredients:

- 1/2 cup pumpkin puree
- 1/2 banana, sliced and frozen
- 1/4 cup pecans (plus more for topping)
- 1/2 teaspoon cinnamon (plus more for topping)
- 1/4 teaspoon nutmeg, 1/4 teaspoon allspice
- 1/8 teaspoon vanilla extract
- 1 cup cashew milk, 1 cup ice
- 1 tablespoon coconut nectar or other liquid sweetener (optional)

Directions:
Combine ingredients in blender and blend until smooth. Pour smoothie into tall glass and serve.

Chocolate, Peanut Butter & Banana Smoothie

Ingredients:

- 12 oz water, milk, or yogurt
- 2 scoops chocolate flavored protein powder
- 1 banana
- 1 cup of spinach
- 2 tbsp of natural peanut butter
- 1 tbsp cacao nibs or dark cocoa powder

Directions:
Combine ingredients in blender and blend until smooth. Pour smoothie into tall glass and serve.

Peanut Butter–Banana Smoothie

Ingredients:

- 1 banana
- 1 cup vanilla yogurt
- 1/2 cup creamy peanut butter
- 1/3 cup milk
- 2 tablespoons malted milk powder
- 1/2 teaspoon cocoa powder
- a pinch of salt
- 2 cups ice

Directions:
Combine ingredients in blender and blend until smooth. Pour smoothie into tall glass and serve.

Banana-Date-Lime Smoothie

Ingredients:

- 2 bananas
- 3/4 cup chopped pitted dates
- 1 lime juice
- 1 1/2 cups each soy milk
- 1 1/2 cups each ice

Directions:
Combine ingredients in blender and blend until smooth. Pour smoothie into tall glass and serve.

Banana Ginger Smoothie

Ingredients:

- 1 banana, sliced
- 3/4 c (6 oz) vanilla yogurt
- 1 Tbsp honey
- 1/2 tsp freshly grated ginger

Directions:
Combine ingredients in blender and blend until smooth. Pour smoothie into tall glass and serve.

Green Spinach Smoothie

Ingredients:

- 1 big handful (about 2/3 bunch) spinach
- 1 handful mint leaves (3 to 4 stems)
- 1/4-inch piece ginger root
- 1/2 banana (fresh or frozen)
- 1/2 cup chunked mango or sliced peaches (fresh or frozen)
- 1/2 cup filtered water

Directions:
Combine ingredients in blender and blend until smooth. Pour smoothie into tall glass and serve.

Banana Pear Smoothie

Ingredients:

- 2 ripe pears, pitted and coarsely chopped
- 1 tsp (5 mL) peeled and coarsely chopped ginger root
- 1 banana
- 1 cup (250 mL) skim milk
- Handful of ice
- Sprinkle of cinnamon on top

Directions:
Combine ingredients in blender and blend until smooth. Pour smoothie into tall glass and serve.

Matcha Smoothie

Ingredients:

- 1 teaspoon matcha green tea powder (no substitutions)
- 2 teaspoons hot water
- 1 cup skim milk
- 1 ripe banana
- 1 tablespoon honey
- 3 to 4 ice cubes

Directions:
Combine ingredients in blender and blend until smooth. Pour smoothie into tall glass and serve.

Honey-Banana Smoothie

Ingredients:

- 1 cup plain non-fat Greek yogurt
- 1 banana
- 1 cup orange juice
- 1 teaspoon honey
- pinch of freshly grated nutmeg

Directions:
Combine ingredients in blender and blend until smooth. Pour smoothie into tall glass and serve.

Peanut Butter-Banana Honey Smoothie

Ingredients:

- 1 cup plain low-fat yogurt
- 1 teaspoon honey
- 1 teaspoon vanilla extract
- 1 cup sliced frozen bananas
- 2 tablespoons peanut butter
- 1/4 cup ice

Directions:
Combine ingredients in blender and blend until smooth. Pour smoothie into tall glass and serve.

Banana Spice Smoothie

Ingredients:

- 2 ripe bananas
- 2 cups vanilla kefir
- 1/2 teaspoon ground cinnamon
- 1/8 teaspoon ground nutmeg
- 1/8 teaspoon ground allspice
- 12 ice cubes

Directions:

Combine ingredients in blender and blend until smooth. Pour smoothie into tall glass and serve.

Banana & Nutty Mango Smoothie

Ingredients:

- 1 cup orange juice
- 1/2 cup natural probiotic yogurt
- 2 mango cheeks
- 1 banana
- Small handful of oats
- 1 tbsp almond butter

Directions:
Combine ingredients in blender and blend until smooth. Pour smoothie into tall glass and serve.

Chocolate-Banana Smoothie

Ingredients:

- 1 frozen banana
- 3/4 cup milk
- 3 tbsp. chocolate syrup
- 3 ice cubes

Directions:
Combine ingredients in blender and blend until smooth. Pour smoothie into tall glass and serve.

Chocolate-Peanut Butter Smoothie

Ingredients:

- 1/2 cup 1% low-fat milk
- 2 tablespoons chocolate syrup
- 2 tablespoons creamy peanut butter
- 1 frozen sliced ripe banana
- 1 (8-ounce) carton vanilla low-fat yogurt

Directions:

Combine ingredients in blender and blend until smooth. Pour smoothie into tall glass and serve.

Pumpkin Pie-Banana Smoothie

Ingredients:

- 1 cup almond milk
- 1/2 cup canned pumpkin puree
- 1 teaspoon pumpkin pie spice
- 1 teaspoon blackstrap molasses
- 1/2 frozen banana or 1/2 scoop vanilla protein powder
- 3 ice cubes

Directions:
Combine ingredients in blender and blend until smooth. Pour smoothie into tall glass and serve.

Almond Butter & Jelly Smoothie

Ingredients:

- 3/4 cup almond milk
- 1 tablespoon almond butter
- 1/2 scoop vanilla protein powder
- 1/2 frozen banana
- 1 tablespoon jam
- 2 tablespoons plain Greek yogurt
- 1/2 teaspoon vanilla extract
- 3 ice cubes

Directions:
Combine ingredients in blender and blend until smooth. Pour smoothie into tall glass and serve.

Orange & Banana Breakfast Smoothie

Ingredients:

- 3/4 cup (185 ml) orange juice
- 1/2 cup sliced banana
- 2 teaspoons brown sugar
- 1/8 teaspoon almond extract
- 2 ice cubes
- Mint sprig

Directions:
Combine ingredients in blender and blend until smooth. Pour smoothie into tall glass and serve.

Tomato Smoothie

Ingredients:

- 225g low-fat plain yogurt
- 2 large ripe plum or round tomatoes, peeled, seeded and chopped
- 1/2 teaspoon dried basil
- 1/2 teaspoon salt cherry tomatoes and ice, to serve (optional)

Directions:
Combine ingredients in blender and blend until smooth. Pour smoothie into tall glass and serve.

Beet & Strawberry Smoothie

Ingredients:

- 4 beets, cooked and peeled
- 2 cups (500 mL) unsweetened coconut water
- 2 cups (500 mL) frozen strawberries
- 1 lime, juiced

Directions:
Combine ingredients in blender and blend until smooth. Pour smoothie into tall glass and serve.

Raspberry-Beet Smoothie

Ingredients:

- 150g cooked beetroots, coarsely chopped
- 60g fresh or frozen raspberries
- 250ml cranberry juice, chilled
- 225g low-fat plain yogurt
- Chilled raspberries, to garnish (optional)

Directions:
Combine ingredients in blender and blend until smooth. Pour smoothie into tall glass and serve.

Carrot-Berry Smoothie

Ingredients:

- 1/2 cup almond milk
- 1/2 cup water
- 1 carrot
- 2 cups spinach
- 1/2 cup frozen berries
- 1 tablespoon chia seeds
- 1 tablespoon hemp protein
- 1/2 teaspoon stevia

Directions:
Combine ingredients in blender and blend until smooth. Pour smoothie into tall glass and serve.

Green Berry Smoothie

Ingredients:

- 1 cup water
- 1 tablespoon chia seeds
- 1/2 cup frozen raspberries
- 1/2 cup frozen wild blueberries
- 1 large handful spinach leaves
- 15 drops organic liquid stevia or 1 stevia packet (optional)

Directions:
Combine ingredients in blender and blend until smooth. Pour smoothie into tall glass and serve.

Cashew Butter Baby Smoothie

Ingredients:

- 1 cup almond milk
- 1/2 cup strawberries
- 1/2 cup raspberries
- 1/4 cup coconut milk, frozen into ice cubes
- 2 tablespoons cashew butter
- 1 tablespoon raw cacao nibs
- 1/2 cup ice

Directions:
Combine ingredients in blender and blend until smooth. Pour smoothie into tall glass and serve.

Wild Blueberry Soy Smoothie

Ingredients:

- 2 cups wild blueberries, frozen
- 1 1/2 cups vanilla soy milk
- 4 tablespoons honey
- 1 dash freshly ground nutmeg
- Garnish with fresh mint leaves

Directions:
Combine ingredients in blender and blend until smooth. Pour smoothie into tall glass and serve.

Citrus Berry Smoothie

Ingredients:

- 1 1/4 cups fresh berries
- 3/4 cup low-fat plain yogurt
- 1/2 cup orange juice
- 2 tablespoons nonfat dry milk
- 1 tablespoon toasted wheat germ
- 1 tablespoon honey
- 1/2 teaspoon vanilla extract

Directions:
Combine ingredients in blender and blend until smooth. Pour smoothie into tall glass and serve.

Kiwi-Strawberry Smoothie

Ingredients:

- 1 cup strawberries
- 2 peeled kiwis
- 2 tablespoons sugar
- 2 cups ice

Directions:
Combine ingredients in blender and blend until smooth. Pour smoothie into tall glass and serve.

Watermelon Bliss Smoothie

Ingredients:

- 2 cups (500 mL) chopped seedless watermelon
- 1 cup (250 mL) strawberries
- 1 cup (250 mL) plain low-fat yogurt
- Handful of ice

Directions:
Combine ingredients in blender and blend until smooth. Pour smoothie into tall glass and serve.

Raspberry Smoothie

Ingredients:

- 1 cup milk
- 1/2 cup orange juice
- 3 oz. silken tofu
- 1 1/2 cup frozen raspberries

Directions:
Combine ingredients in blender and blend until smooth. Pour smoothie into tall glass and serve.

Strawberry Shortcake Smoothie

Ingredients:

- 2 cups strawberries
- 1 cup crumbled pound cake
- 1 1/2 cups each milk and ice
- Sugar to taste
- Top with whipped cream and more strawberries

Directions:
Combine ingredients in blender and blend until smooth. Pour smoothie into tall glass and serve.

Very Berry Super Smoothie

Ingredients:

- 12 oz water
- 1 cup spinach
- 2 cups frozen mixed berries
- 1/2 cup plain low-fat yogurt
- 2 scoops vanilla protein powder
- 1 tbsp walnuts
- 1 tbsp ground flaxseed

Directions:
Combine ingredients in blender and blend until smooth. Pour smoothie into tall glass and serve.

Berry Smoothie

Ingredients:

- 1 cup cranberry juice
- 1 cup frozen blueberries or 1 cup frozen strawberries
- 1 (8 ounce) container vanilla yogurt
- ⅔ cup uncooked oats
- 1 cup ice cube

Directions:
Combine ingredients in blender and blend until smooth. Pour smoothie into tall glass and serve.

Strawberry Yogurt Smoothie

Ingredients:

- 4 cups (1 L) ripe strawberries
- 1 cup (250 mL) plain low-fat yogurt
- 1/2 cup (125 mL) fresh orange juice
- 1 tbsp (15 mL) sugar, or to taste
- Garnish (optional):
- 4 small strawberries with leaves
- 4 thin round slices of unpeeled orange

Directions:
Combine ingredients in blender and blend until smooth. Pour smoothie into tall glass and serve.

Strawberry-Yogurt Smoothie

Ingredients:

- 1 quart (4 cups) ripe strawberries
- 1 cup plain yogurt
- 1/2 cup fresh orange juice
- 1 tablespoon sugar
- 4 thin orange slices (optional)

Directions:
Combine ingredients in blender and blend until smooth. Pour smoothie into tall glass and serve.

Blueberry-Orange Yogurt Smoothie

Ingredients:

- 3 or 4 ice cubes, optional
- 1 cup plain low-fat yogurt
- 1 cup fresh orange juice
- 1 cup fresh or frozen blueberries (if frozen, omit ice cubes)
- 1/2 teaspoon vanilla extract

Directions:
Combine ingredients in blender and blend until smooth. Pour smoothie into tall glass and serve.

Summer Stone Fruit Smoothie

Ingredients:

- 1/2 cup Greek yogurt
- 1 plum, pit removed, flesh roughly chopped
- 1 peach, pit removed, flesh roughly chopped
- 1 nectarine, pit removed, flesh roughly chopped
- 1/2 cup blueberries, fresh or frozen

Directions:
Combine ingredients in blender and blend until smooth. Pour smoothie into tall glass and serve.

Creamsicle Smoothie

Ingredients:

- 2 cups cantaloupe, chunks
- 1 cup orange juice
- 1 tablespoon honey
- 1 teaspoon vanilla
- Ice cube (to thicken) (optional)

Directions:
Combine ingredients in blender and blend until smooth. Pour smoothie into tall glass and serve.

Orange Peach Smoothie

Ingredients:

- 2 cups frozen peach slices
- 1 cup carrot juice
- 1 cup orange juice
- 2 tablespoons ground flaxseed
- 1 tablespoon chopped fresh ginger

Directions:
Combine ingredients in blender and blend until smooth. Pour smoothie into tall glass and serve.

Citrus Energy-Boosting Smoothie

Ingredients:

- 1 orange, peeled and chopped, seeds removed
- 1 lemon, peeled and chopped, seeds removed
- 4 spinach leaves
- 2 carrots, peeled and chopped (or grated)
- 1 1/2 cup (375 mL) almond milk
- 1 peach, peeled and chopped

Directions:
Combine ingredients in blender and blend until smooth. Pour smoothie into tall glass and serve.

Chocolate Cherry Smoothie

Ingredients:

- 12 oz water, milk, or yogurt
- 2 scoops chocolate flavored protein powder
- 2 cups of sweet dark cherries, pits removed
- 1 cups of spinach
- 1 tbsp of walnuts
- 1 tbsp ground flax
- 1 tbsp cacao nibs or dark cocoa powder

Directions:
Combine ingredients in blender and blend until smooth. Pour smoothie into tall glass and serve.

Pomegranate-Cherry Smoothie

Ingredients:

- 1 cup frozen pitted cherries
- 3/4 cup pomegranate juice
- 1/2 cup plain yogurt
- 1 tablespoon honey
- 1 teaspoon lemon juice
- a pinch each of cinnamon and salt
- 2 cups ice

Directions:
Combine ingredients in blender and blend until smooth. Pour smoothie into tall glass and serve.

Vanilla Pumpkin Pie Smoothie

Ingredients:

- 12 oz water, milk, or yogurt
- 2 scoops vanilla flavored protein powder
- 3/4 cup of pureed pumpkin
- 1 tbsp of walnuts
- 1 tbsp of ground flax
- 1/2 cup of uncooked oats
- Cinnamon and vanilla extract to taste
- Ice as needed

Directions:
Combine ingredients in blender and blend until smooth. Pour smoothie into tall glass and serve.

Spinach, Grape & Coconut Smoothie

Ingredients:

- 1cup seedless green grapes
- 1cup packed baby spinach
- 1/2cup ice
- 1/4cup coconut milk

Directions:
Combine ingredients in blender and blend until smooth. Pour smoothie into tall glass and serve.

Double Chocolate Mint Smoothie

Ingredients:

- 1 scoop chocolate protein powder
- 3/4 cup Silk Almond milk, dark chocolate
- 1 tbsp walnuts
- 2 tbsp cocoa powder, unsweetened
- 1 tbsp cacao nibs
- 2 mint leaves
- 4 ice cubes
- 1/4 cup water

Directions:
Combine ingredients in blender and blend until smooth. Pour smoothie into tall glass and serve.

Coconut Almond Smoothie

Ingredients:

- 1 scoop chocolate protein powder
- 1 tbsp unsweetened coconut flakes
- 1 cup Silk Almond milk, dark chocolate
- 1 rounded tbsp almond butter
- 1 1/2 cups water
- 3 ice cubes

Directions:
Combine ingredients in blender and blend until smooth. Pour smoothie into tall glass and serve.

Chocolate Peanut Butter Smoothie

Ingredients:

- 2 tbsp flaxmeal
- 1 tbsp unsweetened cocoa powder
- 1 tbsp natural peanut butter
- 1 scoop chocolate whey protein powder
- Water as needed

Directions:
Combine ingredients in blender and blend until smooth. Pour smoothie into tall glass and serve.

Cappuccino Smoothies

Ingredients:

- 2 tablespoons instant coffee crystals
- 2 tablespoons hot water
- 2 cups premium vanilla ice cream
- ¼ cup instant powdered chocolate milk mix
- 1 ½ cups milk

Directions:
Combine ingredients in blender and blend until smooth. Pour smoothie into tall glass and serve.

Clean Breeze Smoothie

Ingredients:

- 1 small cucumber, chopped
- 2 ripe kiwis, peeled
- 1 cup ginger-flavored kombucha
- 1/2 cup low-fat plain Greek yogurt
- 2 tablespoons fresh cilantro leaves
- 6 ice cubes

Directions:
Combine ingredients in blender and blend until smooth. Pour smoothie into tall glass and serve.

Almond-Orange Smoothie

Ingredients:

- 1 cup (250 mL) vanilla-flavored almond beverage
- 1/2 cup (125 mL) orange juice
- Juice from one lemon
- Juice from one lime
- Handful of ice
- 1 Tbsp (15 mL) honey

Directions:
Combine ingredients in blender and blend until smooth. Pour smoothie into tall glass and serve.

Honeydew-Almond Smoothie

Ingredients:

- 2 cups chopped honeydew melon
- 1 cup almond milk
- 1 cup ice
- Honey to taste

Directions:
Combine ingredients in blender and blend until smooth. Pour smoothie into tall glass and serve.

Oatmeal Cookie Smoothie

Ingredients:

- 1 cup each vanilla ice cream
- 1 cup milk
- 1 cup crumbled oatmeal cookies
- A pinch of ground cinnamon

Directions:
Combine ingredients in blender and blend until smooth. Pour smoothie into tall glass and serve.

Spiced Pumpkin Smoothie

Ingredients:

- 1/2 cup pumpkin puree
- 1/2 cup silken tofu
- 3 1/2 tablespoons brown sugar
- 1 cup milk
- 1/2 teaspoon pumpkin pie spice
- a pinch of salt
- 1 cup ice

Directions:
Combine ingredients in blender and blend until smooth. Pour smoothie into tall glass and serve.

Chocolate Chip Cookie Smoothie

Ingredients:

- 1 cup vanilla ice cream
- 1 cup milk
- 1 cup crumbled chocolate chip cookies
- 1/4 cup mini chocolate chips
- Top with a cookie.

Directions:
Combine ingredients in blender and blend until smooth. Pour smoothie into tall glass and serve.

Orange Creamsicle Smoothie

Ingredients:

- 1 scoop vanilla protein powder
- 1 orange
- 1/4 orange peel
- 1 tbsp walnuts
- 2 tbsp flaxseed meal
- 1 cup water
- 1/2 cup orange juice
- 3 ice cubes

Directions:
Combine ingredients in blender and blend until smooth. Pour smoothie
into tall glass and serve.

Orange Dream Creamsicle Smoothie

Ingredients:

- 1 navel orange, peeled
- 1/4 c fat-free half-and-half or fat-free yogurt
- 2 Tbsp frozen orange juice concentrate
- 1/4 tsp vanilla extract
- 4 ice cubes

Directions:
Combine ingredients in blender and blend until smooth. Pour smoothie into tall glass and serve.

Watermelon Berry Smoothie

Ingredients:

- 2 cups cubed watermelon
- 1 cup fresh raspberries
- 1 cup frozen blueberries
- 1 cup ice

Directions:
Combine ingredients in blender and blend until smooth. Pour smoothie into tall glass and serve.